D1370311

ONE DAY AT A TIME
CHILDREN LIVING WITH LEUKAEMIA

DON'T
TURN
AWAY

My warmest thanks to Dr Lars Åström and his staff at the children's oncological ward of the Karolinska Hospital for letting me follow their work and the treatment of the children.

British Library Cataloguing in Publication Data
Bergman, Thomas, *1947-*
    One day at a time.
    1. Cancer victims,   - Personal observations
    I. Title II. Series
    362.1'96994'0924

    ISBN 0-83687-064-6
    ISBN 0-83687-060-3 series

D O N 'T
T U R N
A W A Y

United Kingdom edition first published in 1989 by

Gareth Stevens Children's Books
31 Newington Green
London N16 9PU

Series Editor: MaryLee Knowlton
Research Editor: Scott Enk
Series Designer: Kate Kriege

Printed in the United States of America

1 2 3 4 5 6 7 8 9 95 94 93 92 91 90 89

ONE DAY AT A TIME

CHILDREN LIVING WITH LEUKAEMIA

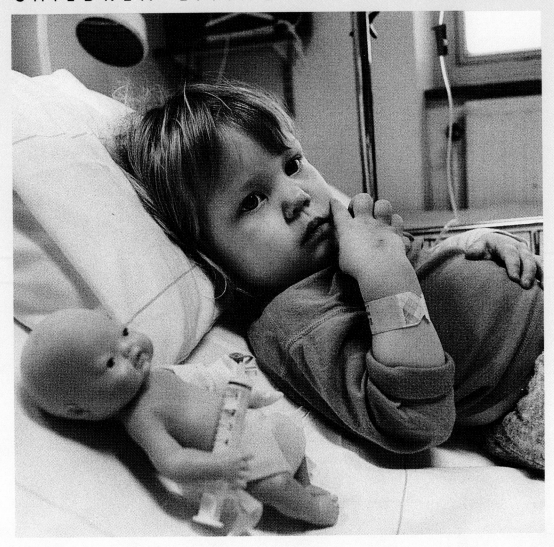

DON'T
TURN
AWAY

Thomas Bergman

Gareth Stevens Children's Books
LONDON • MILWAUKEE

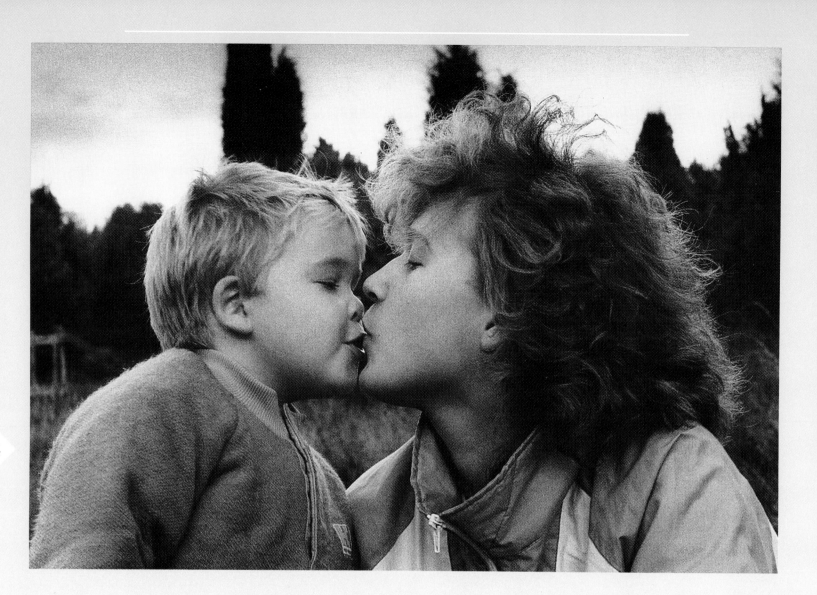

When Thomas Bergman first showed me the remarkable photographs that appear in One Day at a Time, I was struck by their power to capture the essence of children's personalities and moods. As we looked at them together — I for the first time, he once again after many times — I was moved by the intensity and passion of a person who cares deeply about children who are ill.

Thomas is Sweden's best-known children's photographer, with a reputation stretching from Europe to Japan. His compassion, admiration, and affection for children with serious illnesses inspired him to embark on a special photographic mission. The striking black-and-white photographs you will see in this book will remain in your memory. The thoughts and feelings that Thomas's young friends have shared with him form the basis for the text that accompanies the pictures.

You will meet children in the pages of this book with a serious illness that may be unfamiliar to you. You will be inspired by the originality and courage with which they meet the challenges of this illness. You will be moved by the many ways that they are like children everywhere.

In One Day at a Time, Hanna and Frederick show us all that an illness should not be a cause for embarrassment, alienation or fear. Instead, it should be a reason for reaching out, sharing the joys, sorrows, and hopes of our lives.

Gareth Stevens
Gareth Stevens
PUBLISHER

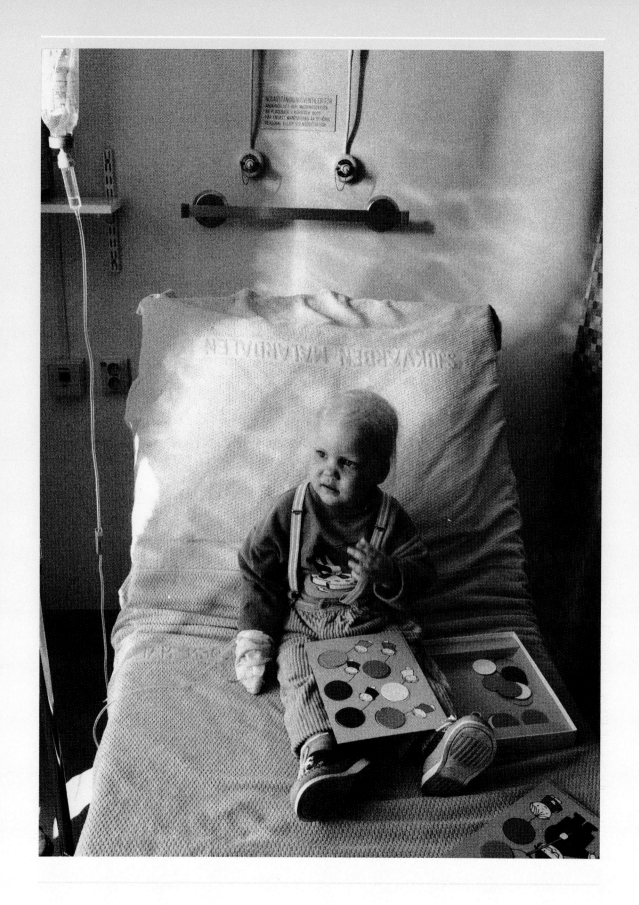

For over twenty years, I have photographed children who have been challenged by life as most of us have not. In that time, I have learned to treasure the special strength that they bring to their struggle and the joy and vibrancy of their lives. The two children you will meet in the pages that follow are very special to me.

Hanna and Frederick have leukaemia. When I met them, Hanna, who is two, was at the very beginning of her disease. Three-year-old Frederick had been ill for six months. For the next eight months, they and their families let me share their experiences, good and bad, and I am pleased to share them now with you.

Before you meet Hanna and Frederick, let me tell you a few things about leukaemia.

Leukaemia is a disease of the blood, a form of cancer. Leukaemia cells grow and multiply in the bone marrow where the blood is produced, destroying and taking the place of normal blood cells. Normal cells have specific jobs to do in the body. When they are destroyed by leukaemia cells, these jobs do not get done and the body begins to fail.

Normal blood is made up of three types of cells — white blood cells, platelets, and red blood cells. When the white blood cells are destroyed, the body cannot fight infections and a simple cold can become life-threatening. Platelets help the blood coagulate. Without them the body cannot control its bleeding. Red blood cells carry oxygen throughout the body. When they are destroyed, the body becomes anaemic, leaving a person weak and exhausted. Leukaemia cells can attack and destroy all three kinds of normal blood cells.

Treatment for children with leukaemia is painful and long. But very often, it is also successful. Over half of the children who get leukaemia will recover completely. As you follow Hanna and Frederick through eight months of their lives, you will learn more about the treatment. You will also learn, as I have, about the courage and love that sustain these children and their parents as they take life as it comes — one day at a time.

Thomas Bergman

Thomas Bergman

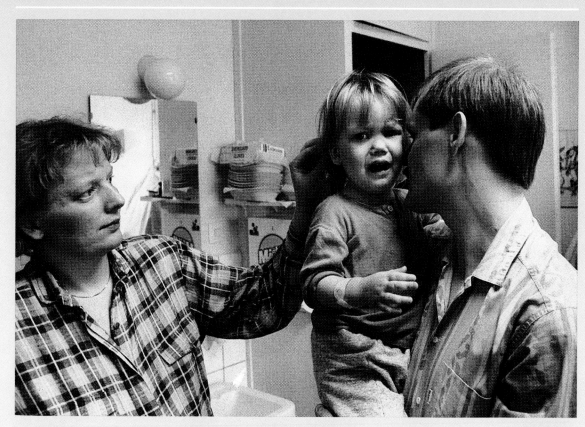

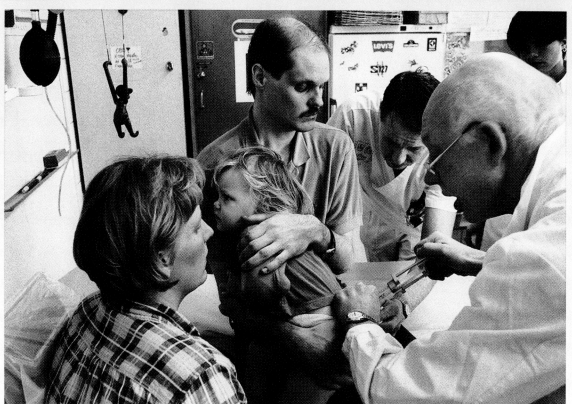

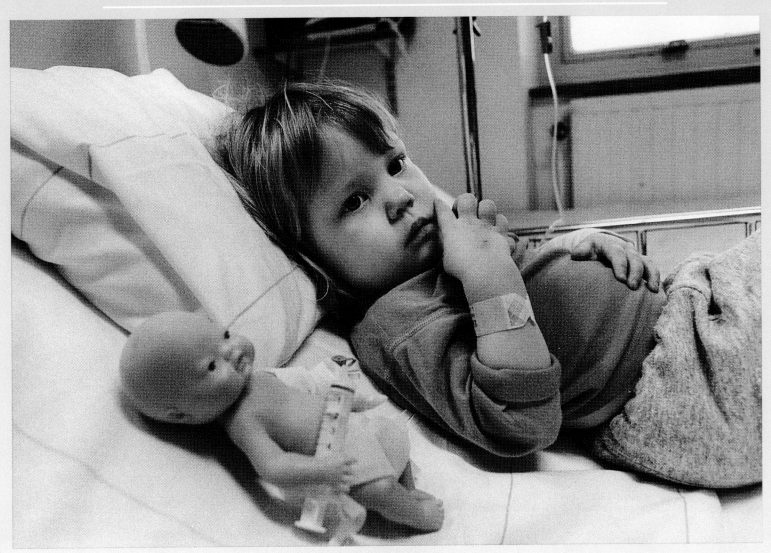

HANNA

Hanna is two years old and has been sick for two weeks with a fever, a cough, and pain in her legs. Blood tests have shown that she suffers from severe anaemia. Hanna is now at the hospital with her mother and father. They now realize that their daughter is seriously ill and are afraid of what is going to happen. The doctor is taking bone marrow from Hanna's hip. He gives her an injection so she won't feel pain. With a syringe, he suctions bone marrow to examine under a microscope. After a while the doctor knows which illness Hanna has. He tells her parents that she has leukaemia, a severe blood disease. It is a form of cancer that can be cured in many children. But not all. Hanna's parents listen intently and become sad. Hanna has a needle in a vein in her arm. Through that needle she will get blood and, tomorrow, medicine. Hanna gives her doll the same treatment.

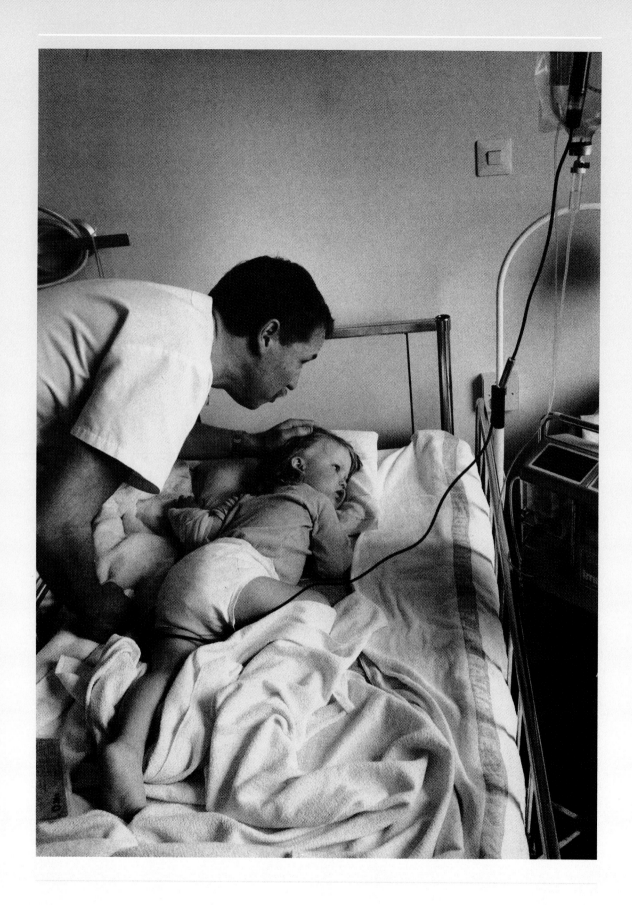

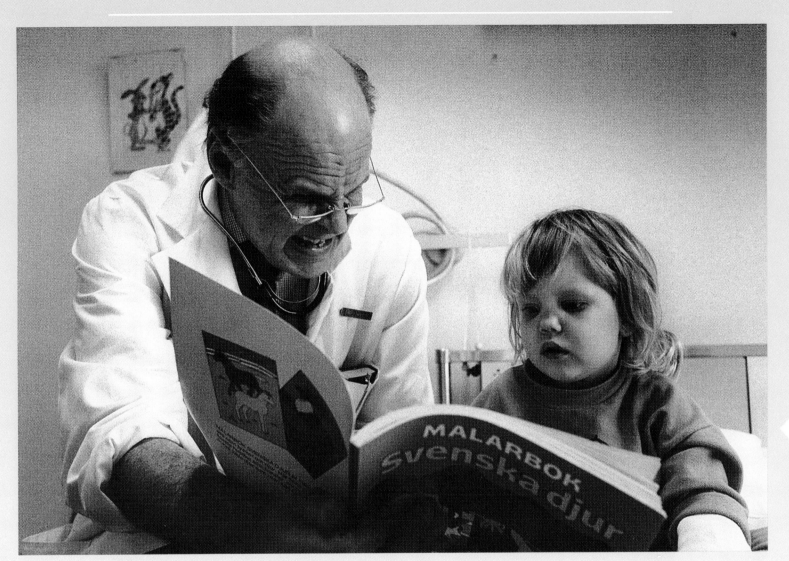

Hanna's mother was pregnant when Hanna became ill. But Hanna was back home when her little brother was born. She is very fond of him. She does not see many other children now because she must not catch a cold. The leukaemia and the treatment have weakened her and a cold could become a serious infection. She misses all her playmates from her nursery school.

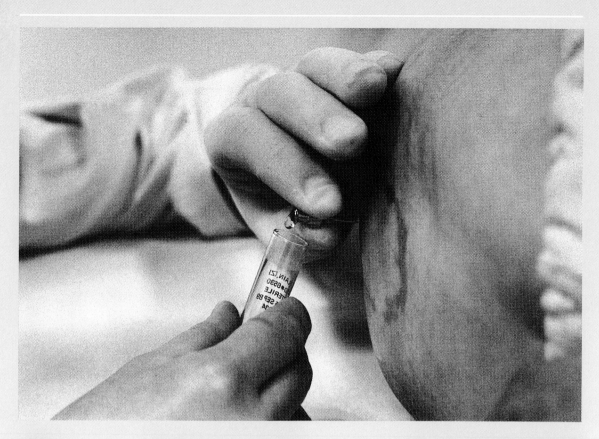

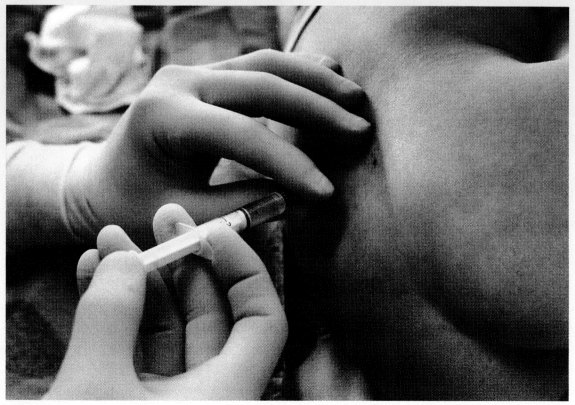

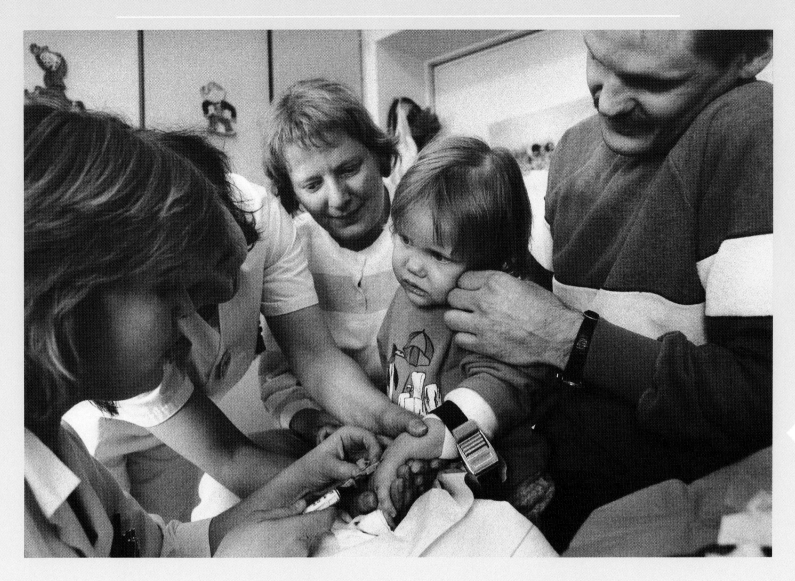

Hanna must have medicine injected into her spinal canal in order to kill
all the leukaemia cells. Her mother and a nurse hold her still while the doctor
gives her an injection. This first one will keep her from feeling pain. Once
it takes effect, the area is numb. Then the doctor puts a needle in her spine.
A liquid like water drips into a test tube. He takes enough for a microscope
examination and then he injects the medicine through the same needle.
Now Hanna must lie very still on her back for one hour to avoid getting a
headache. Then, her nurse takes her to the treatment room to give her new
injections. Hanna receives her first doses of medicine intravenously to kill
the cancer cells in her blood. She is in tears, angry with all the adults who
have held her and hurt her. She does not realize that they had to do this to
help her. They will have to give her more doses of medicine over many
weeks. During the course of the treatment, she is going to lose her hair.

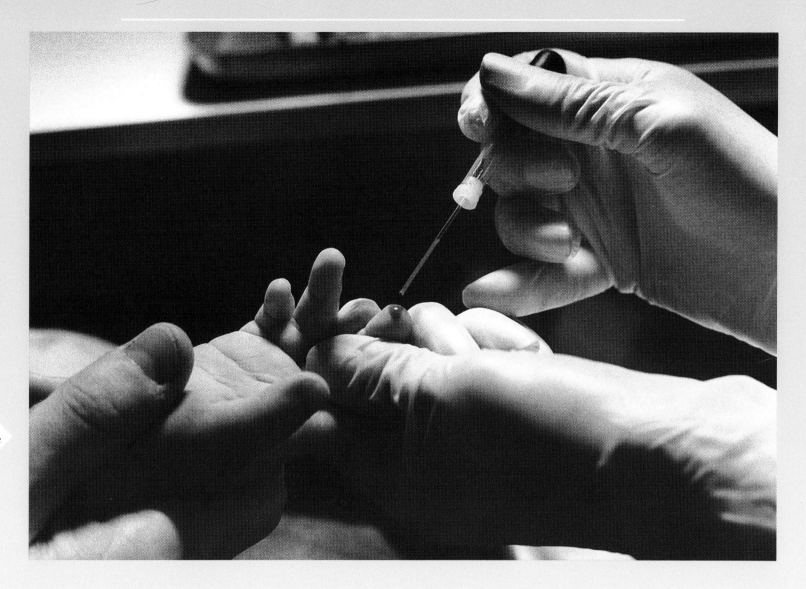

Every morning the nurse comes to take new blood samples. She pricks Hanna's fingertip so that a few drops of blood appear. It hurts just a little and makes Hanna jump, but is soon over. The nurse suctions the blood from the fingertip with a small tube, called a pipette. From the sample, she will find out if Hanna has anaemia. Next she strikes out a drop on a glass slide which she examines with a microscope to see if it contains leukaemia cells. Hanna's blood is not good now. She is still anaemic and her blood still shows leukaemia cells.

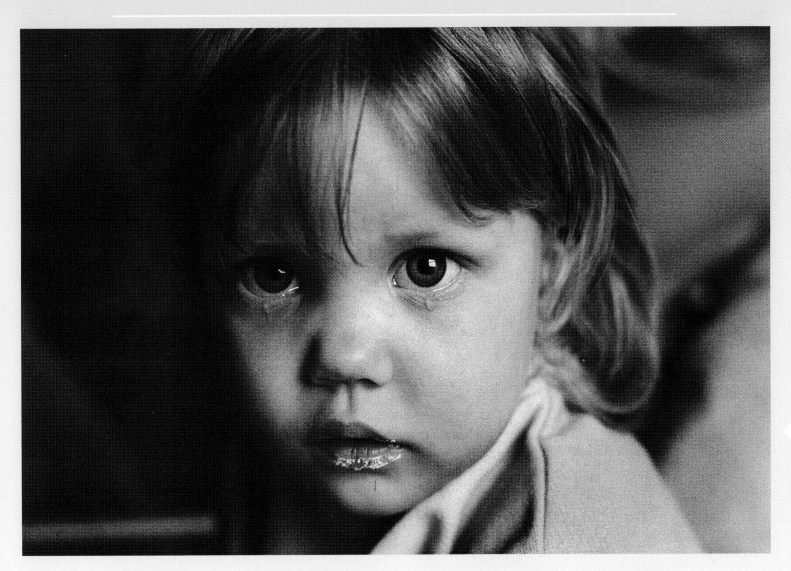

Hanna has been in the hospital for three days. Her parents are allowed to sleep in the room with her. As soon as she wakes up in the morning she turns to her father. 'No more needles, daddy, no more tubes,' she says. Then she turns to her mother. 'I don't like the treatment room. I don't want to go there again.' After just three days she knows what the day will bring. She knows that she will get new injections in the treatment room. She needs her mother and father with her all the time. Then she can get through it.

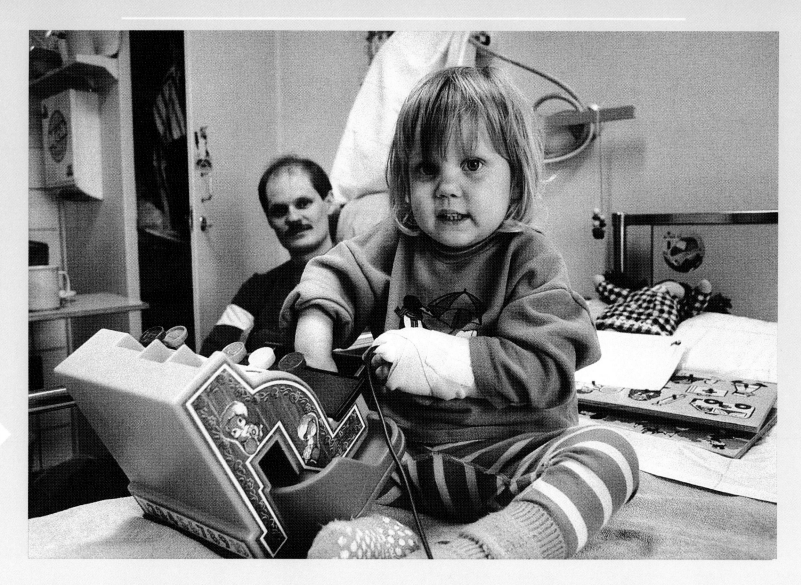

During the first week, Hanna has clung to her parents, never letting them out of her sight. But this afternoon she is more alert and happy and she plays at being a checkout girl. She once again receives a blood transfusion because she still has anaemia.

Hanna has never been ill before. Everything is new and unfamiliar. Hanna wonders if she is going to stay at the hospital for the rest of her life.

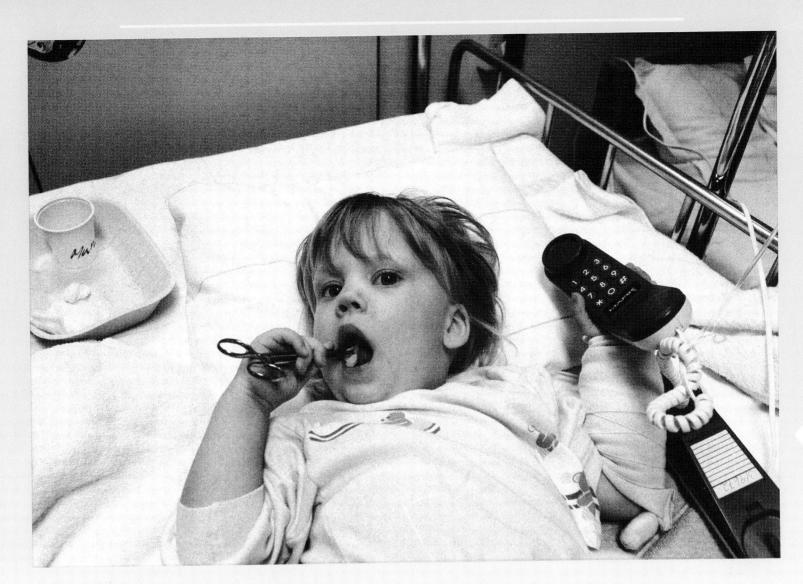

It is difficult to explain to small children why they are sick and cannot be cured at once. At night, when Hanna gets ready for bed, she is not allowed to brush her teeth as usual. Her gums bleed easily because of the disease and the medicines. She has to wash her mouth and can do it by herself.

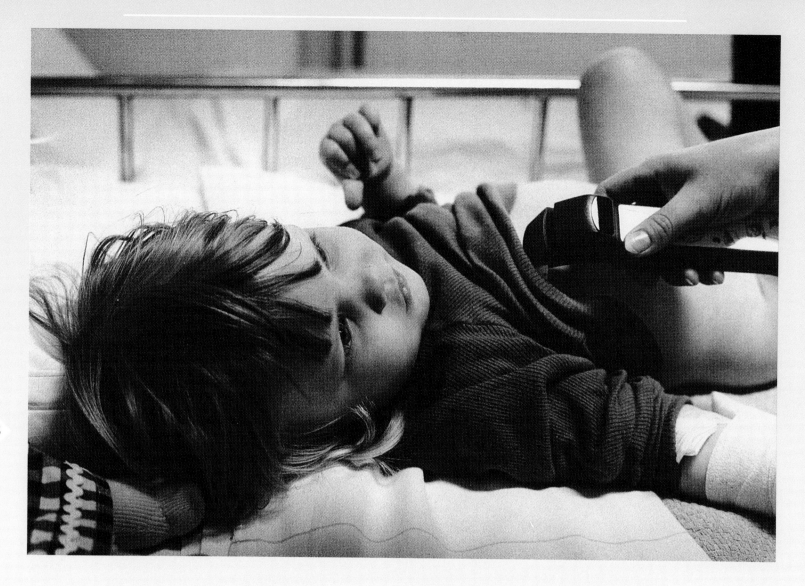

Hanna is very homesick after the long time at the hospital. She longs to get away, to go home. Hanna has been in her room almost all the time. Because she is coughing and has a fever she is not allowed to go to the playroom. She might infect the other children, not with the leukaemia, but with any other infection she might be carrying.

The children's nurse reads Hanna's temperature with a long instrument that looks like a crocodile. Hanna keeps it in her armpit for a minute. It shows that she still has a fever.

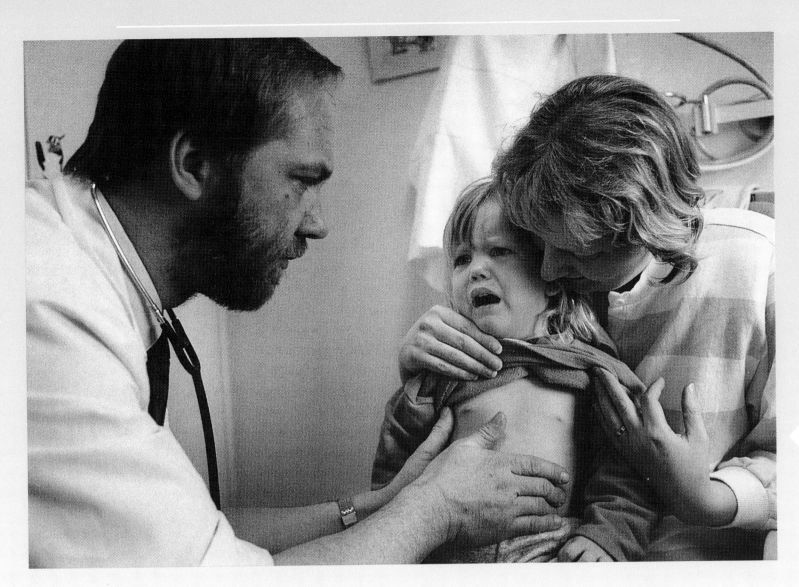

The doctor comes to listen to her lungs and to look in her throat. He gives her medicine to take away the cough and fever. 'In a few days she will feel much better,' he tells her parents.

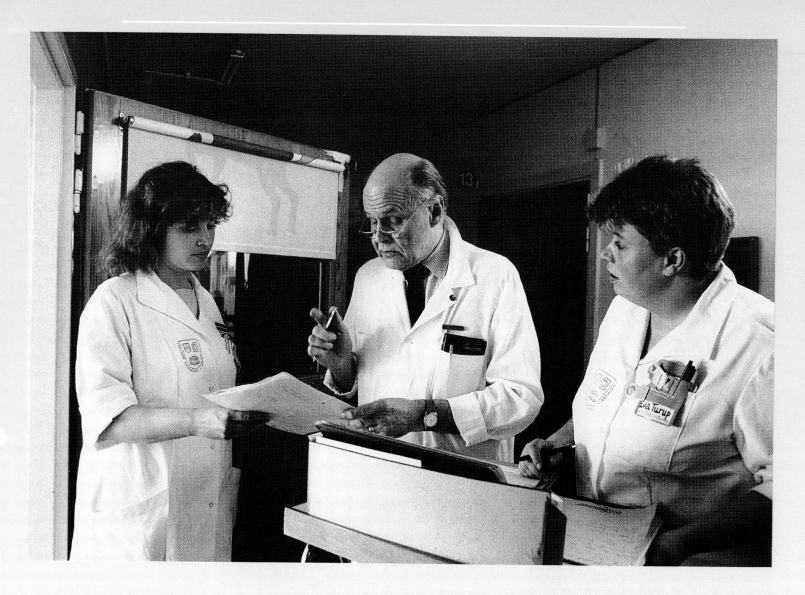

The doctor and the nurse are doing afternoon rounds. Hanna's room is their last stop. The doctor has good news. 'Hanna's blood tests are much better. You can go for a walk in the park. The sun is shining and some fresh air will do her good.' Hanna can now go home for the day and come back to the hospital just to sleep. Soon she will be able to sleep at home.

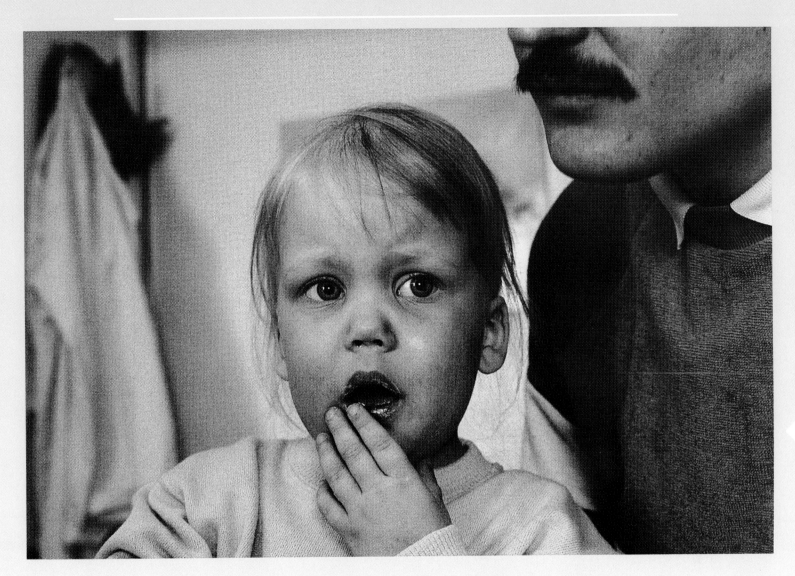

Hanna's parents are thrilled. But after four weeks of anxiety they don't know if they dare to believe what the doctor says. Hanna is already packing her little bag to go home. She believes him.

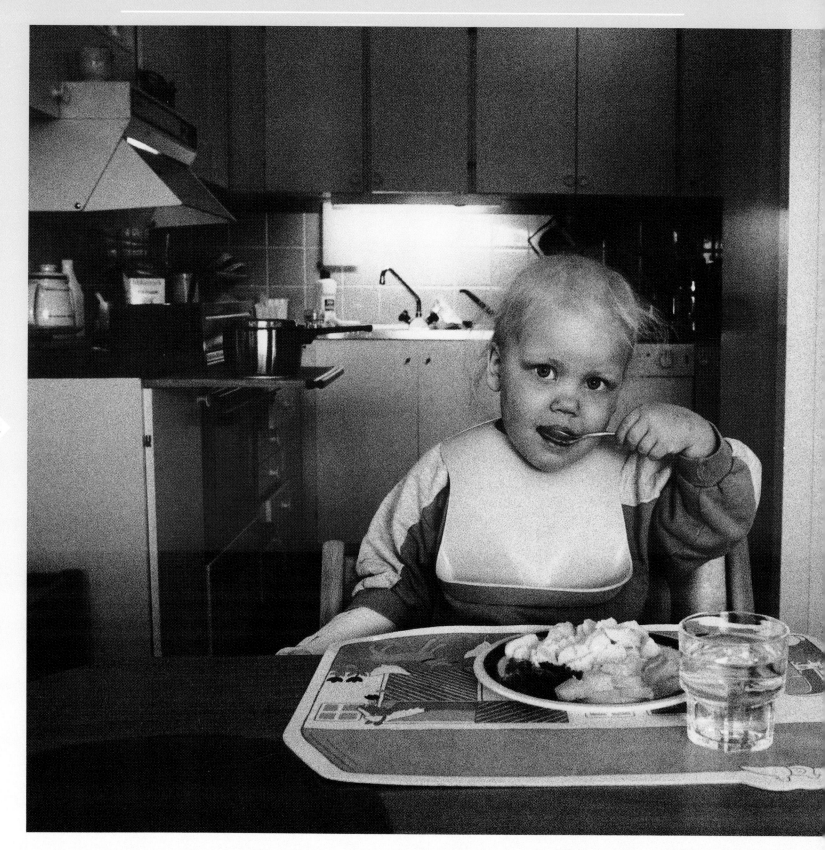

At last Hanna is at home. At night she snuggles into her parents' big, broad bed, just as she did before she became ill. She needs to feel that she really is at home. Her old toys look like old friends.

So many things have happened at the hospital. Now she wants peace and to be in her own room with her teddy bear. Nobody disturbs her. No nurse comes to take blood samples. Best of all, she does not have to go to the treatment room. Hanna shouts, 'I want food, more food!' She eats all afternoon. With her mother's cooking making her feel at home, she takes her medicine by herself.

Later, when Hanna is having her bath, she says, 'I don't want to wash my hair.' Sadly, she has lost almost all her hair.

23

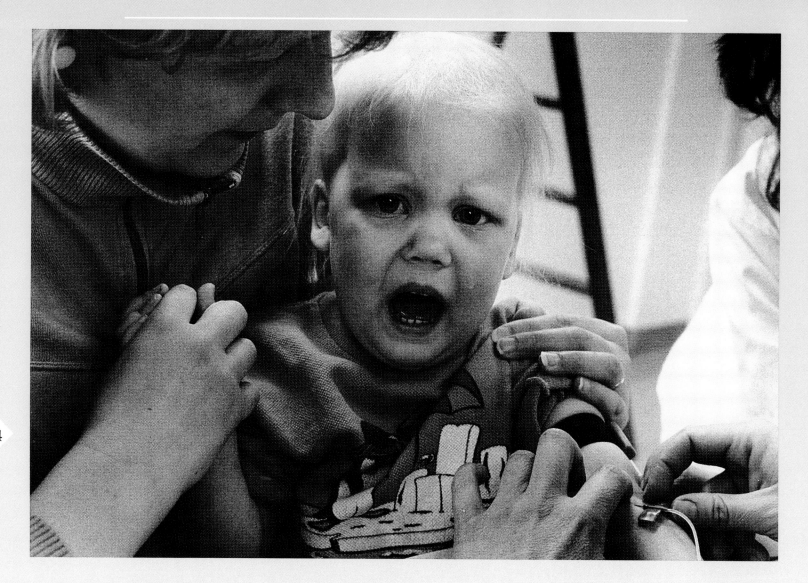

Once a week Hanna goes to the hospital for blood tests which will show immediately if the treatment is working. Hanna is feeling pretty good today and her blood values are improved.

Today, she also gets an injection of medication. The needle looks like a butterfly. Sometimes Hanna is upset when she gets the shot. She wants to hide in her mother's arms. After her shot, she may choose a toy from the 'injection basket'. Today she takes a doll with long, dark hair.

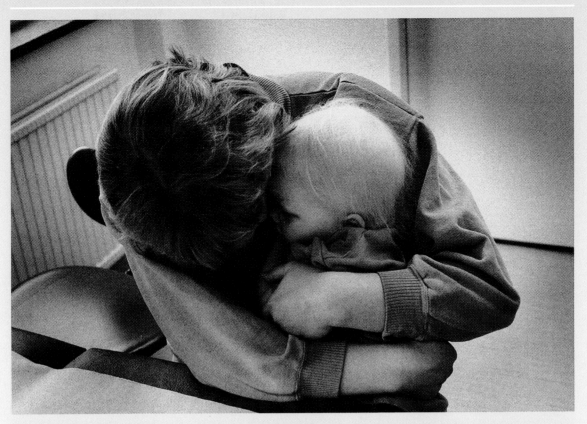

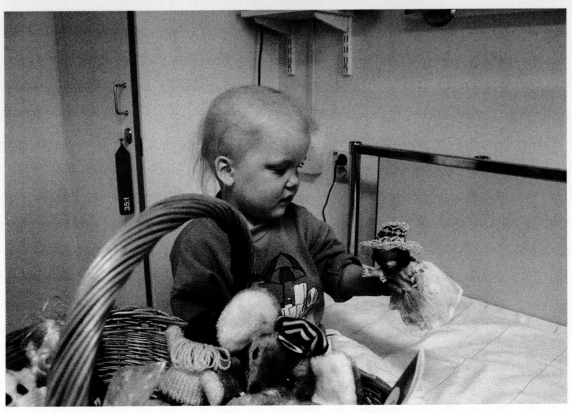

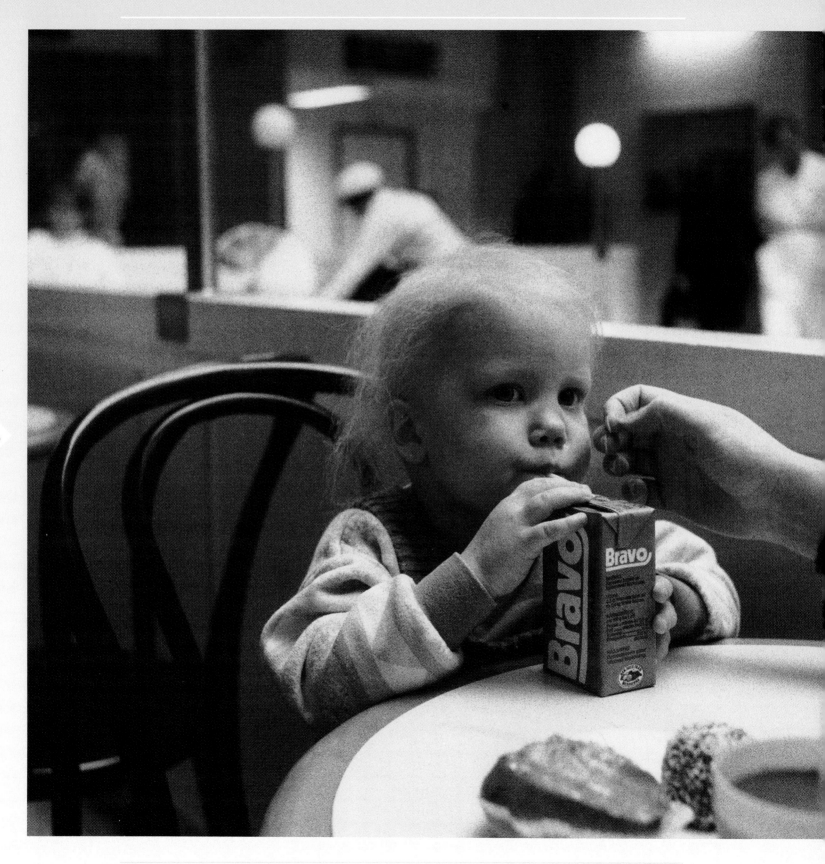

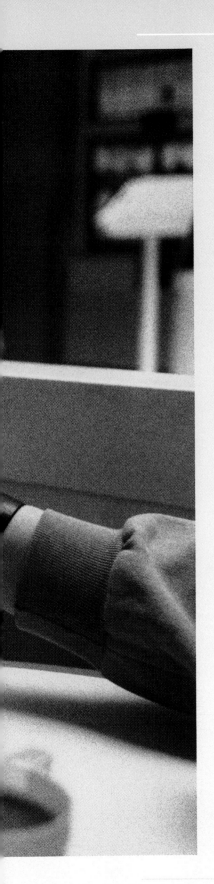

When Hanna's treatment is over, she and her mother visit the coffee shop in the hospital. This is Hanna's favourite part of the day. She has apple juice and cake and her mother has a cup of coffee. It is a nice end to the hospital visit. Hanna is delighted to sit and look at all the people passing through the big entrance. When they have finished, they call a taxi to take them home.

27

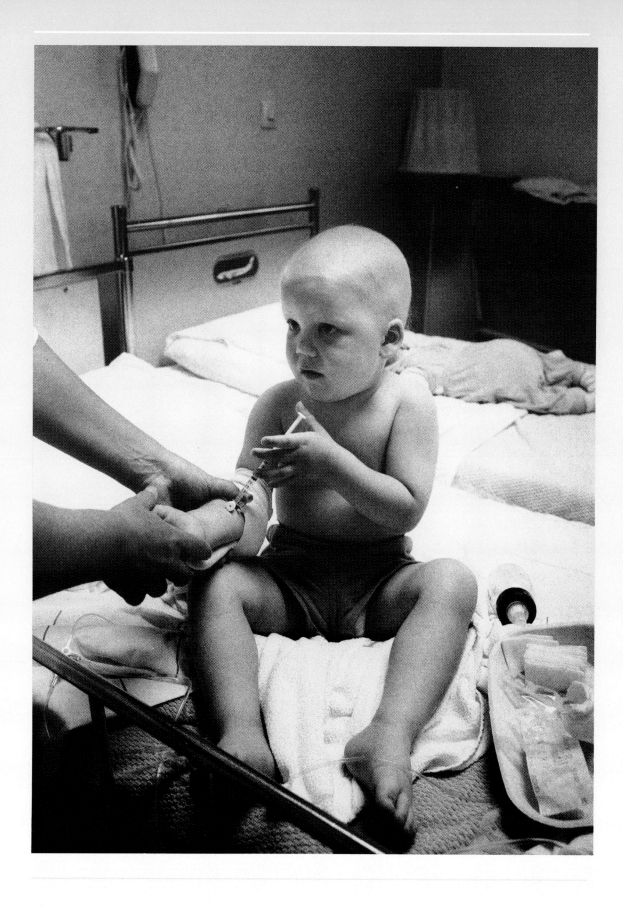

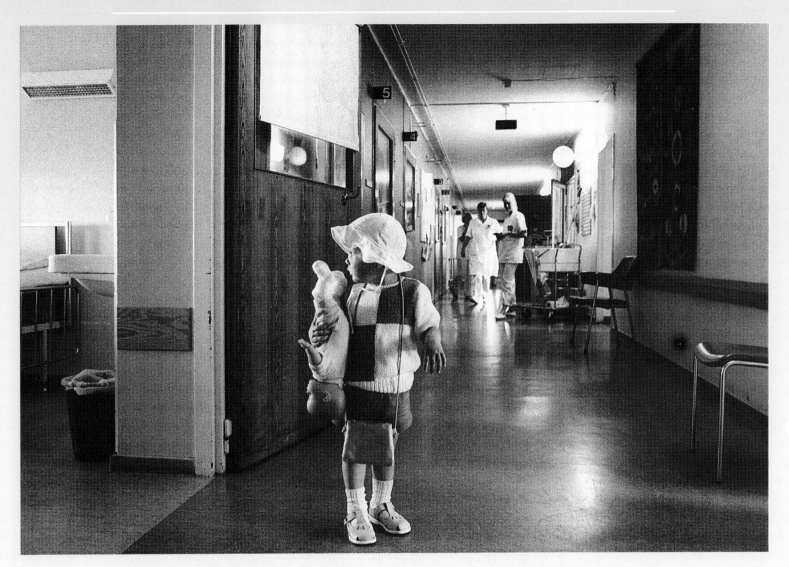

Hanna has now lost all her hair.

She has been at the hospital so often that she is no longer as afraid as
before. This time she and her father have spent the night there. She knows
that she only needs to stay for a few days. She can even give herself an
injection during the treatment. Hanna is curious about the children staying
in the rooms where she has stayed before. She carries her doll around to
all the rooms. She even dares to go to the treatment room, which she was
afraid of earlier, on her own.

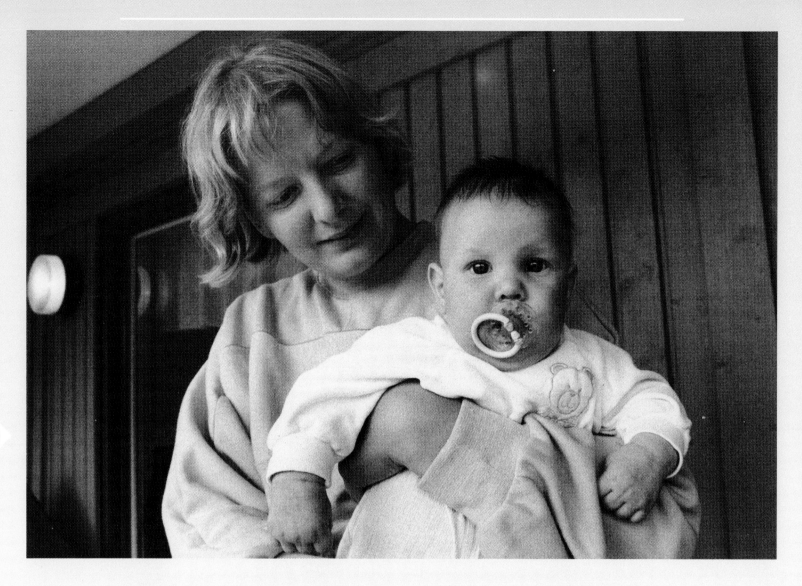

Hanna is tired and pale from her anaemia. Now she gets a blood transfusion to feel better. Kent, a nurse, comes in to look after her and control the blood dripping into her arm. The doctor sits down at Hanna's bed to chat. She is afraid. He wants her to be calm and confident, so he has brought a picture book with different animals which he imitates. Hanna begins to relax. When he asks her the colours of a tiger, she answers, 'Yellow and black, of course, silly.' Some of her fear is forgotten for the moment.

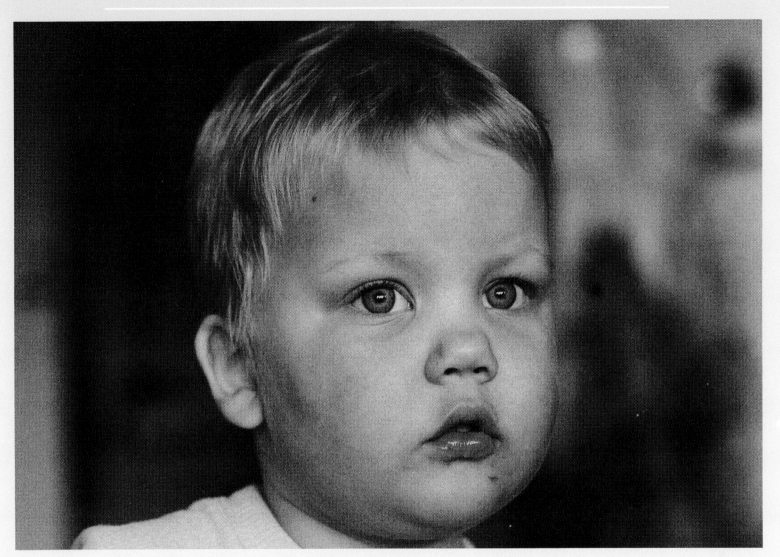

Hanna's parents talk about her illness. 'If Hanna were not so brave and strong, we could not have coped with her disease as well as we have actually done so far. Think of all the pills she has taken! Even though they taste awful, she has swallowed them. The injections she has had throughout her treatment have been very painful. Her tiny veins are like sewing threads. It has often been necessary to prick her several times. She has been hurt and afraid and yet she stretched out her little hand every time.'

Hanna realizes now that all the injections and pills are necessary to cure her, even if nobody knows for sure that they will. She has more than two years of treatment to go through. Her family can only wait and hope for the best. For now, Hanna's hair has grown again. It is lighter than before.

FREDERICK

Frederick is three years old and for six months has had leukaemia, the same disease as Hanna's. Frederick's disease also started with a fever and coughing. Both his legs hurt when he walked. He couldn't play or climb or run around as he had before. He could only take tiny baby steps. He did not eat, either. His mother says, 'We thought he was going to die. But at the hospital they took good care of Frederick. They gave him blood the first three days and he got medicine to kill the leukaemia cells. His treatment will go on for three years. After three weeks he was doing so well that we could go home. Two months later Frederick lost all his hair. But he just said "Oh, look! I'm bald!" He wasn't nearly as upset as we were. But we were sad, not just for his hair, but because of his leukaemia.'

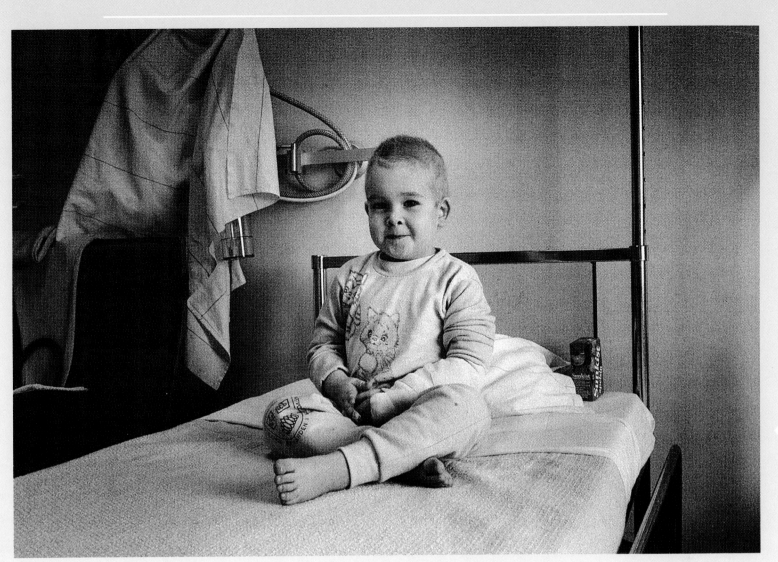

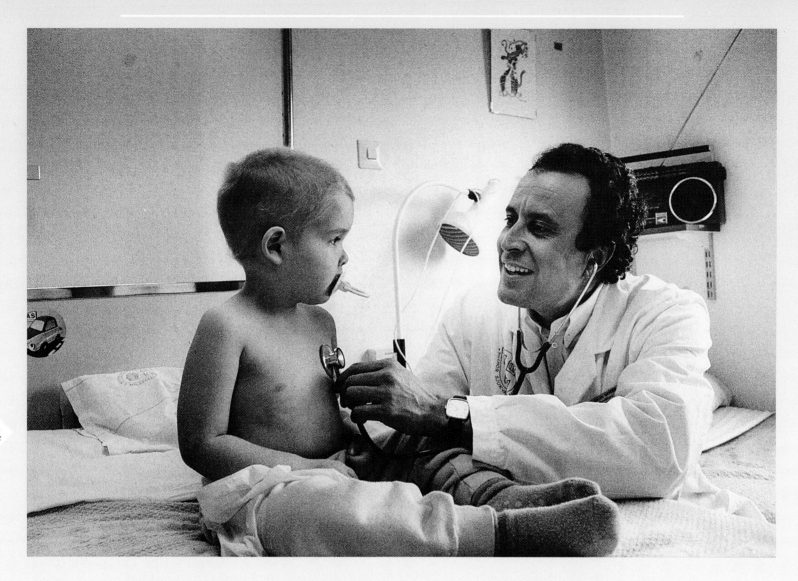

'Daddy, I have to go to the hospital,' Frederick said this morning. 'I don't feel well.' He is calm when he arrives there. He knows that the nurses and doctors will help him when he is ill. The doctor examines him immediately. There are often ups and downs with Frederick's blood values. Now they are bad, so he has frequent nosebleeds, which are very unpleasant. His father says proudly, 'Frederick is brave and fights hard.' He accepts all treatments. Even when the nurse gives him injections that burn and hurt, Frederick tries to hold back his tears. But it hurts too much and he is unhappy and even angry with the nurse.

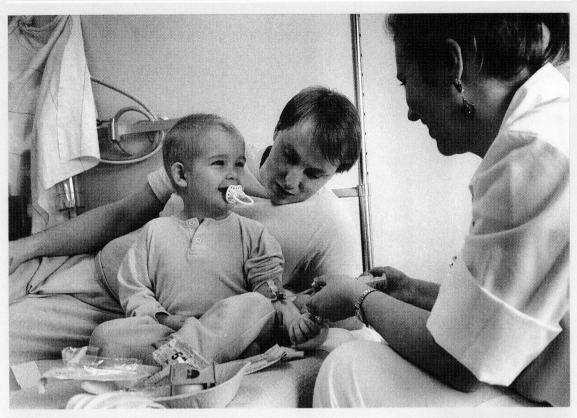

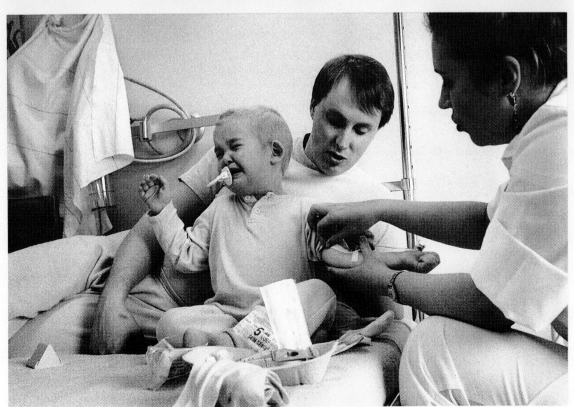

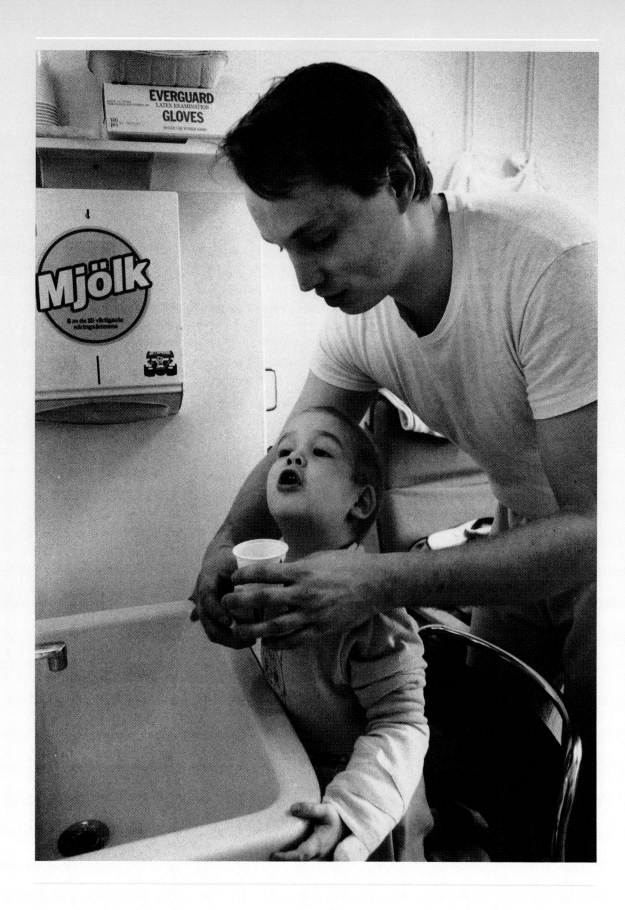

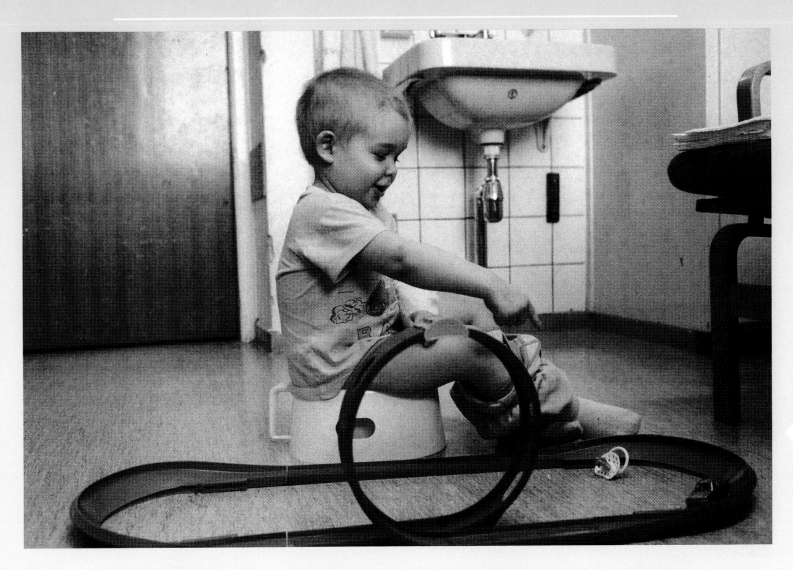

Fortunately, there are treatments which don't hurt, like mouth cleaning. He can manage that all by himself, and it cheers him up. Later Frederick needs a potty-chair. He plays with toys while he sits. Going to the bathroom takes a long time because the medicine gives him stomach problems. He must have his model car track. His father patiently retrieves the cars that Frederick sends flying around the room. Frederick will be in the hospital for ten days this time.

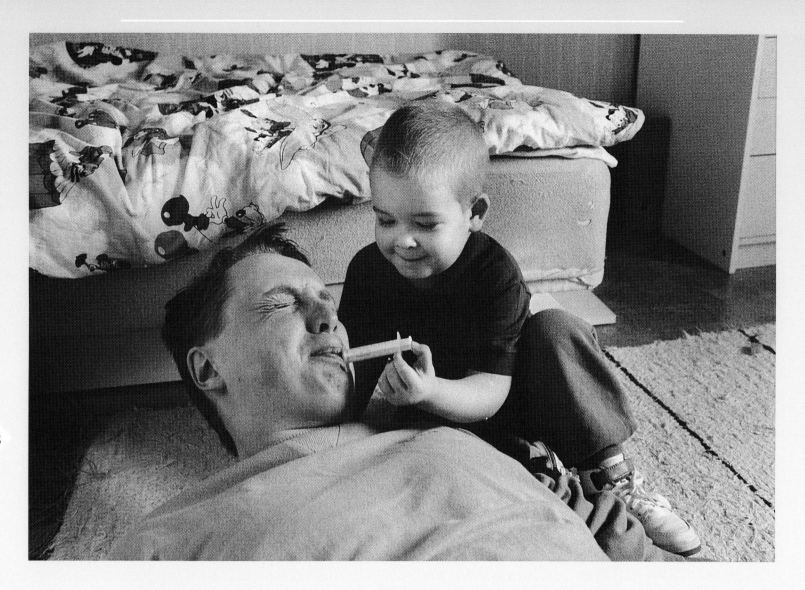

At home Frederick is an active, cheerful little boy. He loves to play with his little brother. They often play hospital games. Frederick gives 'injections' to both his parents and to his brother. After a while, his brother is tired of getting 'injections'. So his father has to have some more, both in his arms and in his mouth. Frederick likes to lie under the sun lamp because of the funny sunglasses he must wear there.

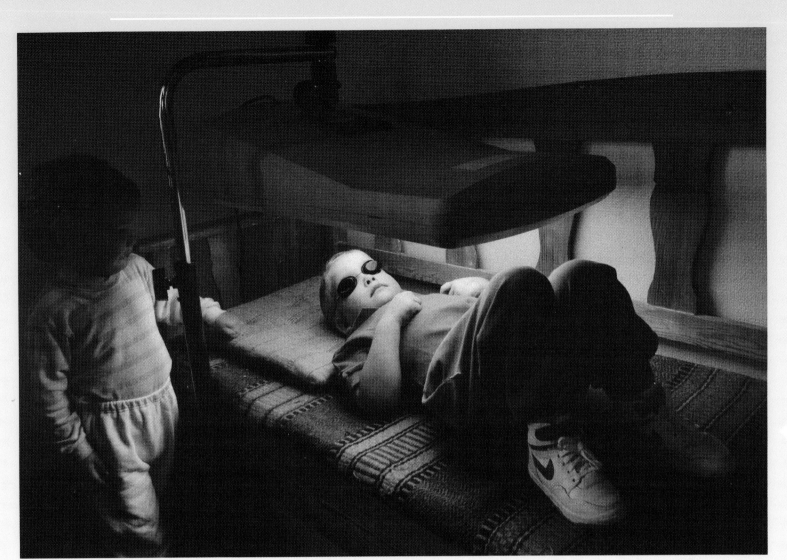

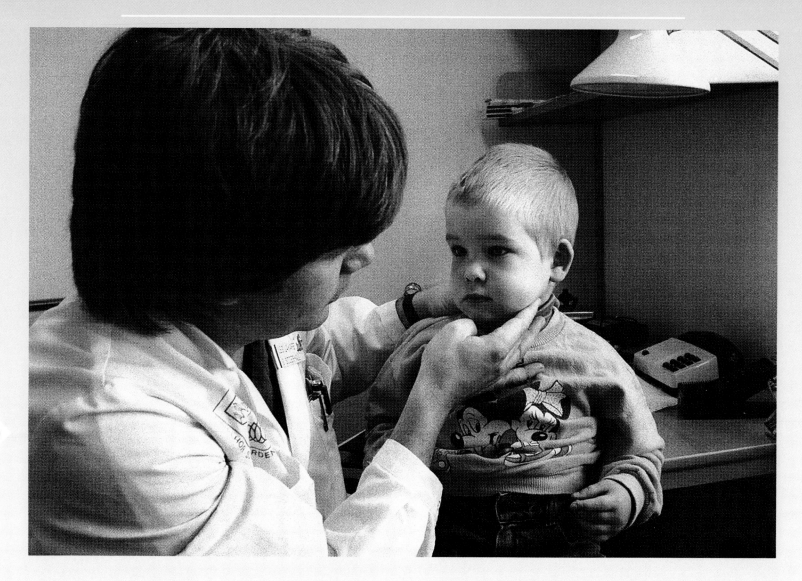

Once a week Frederick goes to the hospital for a checkup. Each time he sees a doctor he knows well. Three doctors work at the ward for children with cancer. Frederick's parents can always call one of them if Frederick is ill at home. They can reach a doctor even at night if necessary. It is very important that the whole family have confidence in the staff who work with Frederick. They talk not only about the disease but also about how the whole family feels.

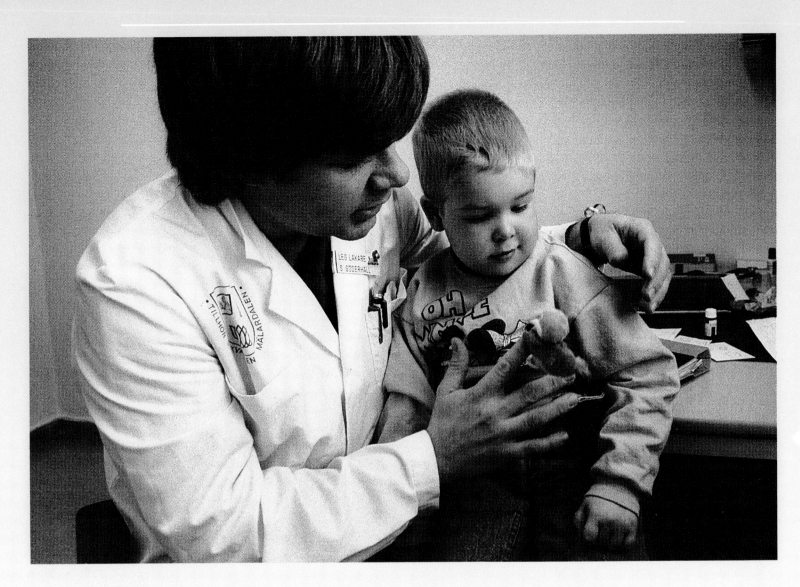

Sometimes Frederick shouts angrily without any reason, which is very frustrating for his parents. The doctor tells them that one of Frederick's medicines often makes the children angry and impatient. They adjust his medication schedule so he doesn't have to take that one all the time.

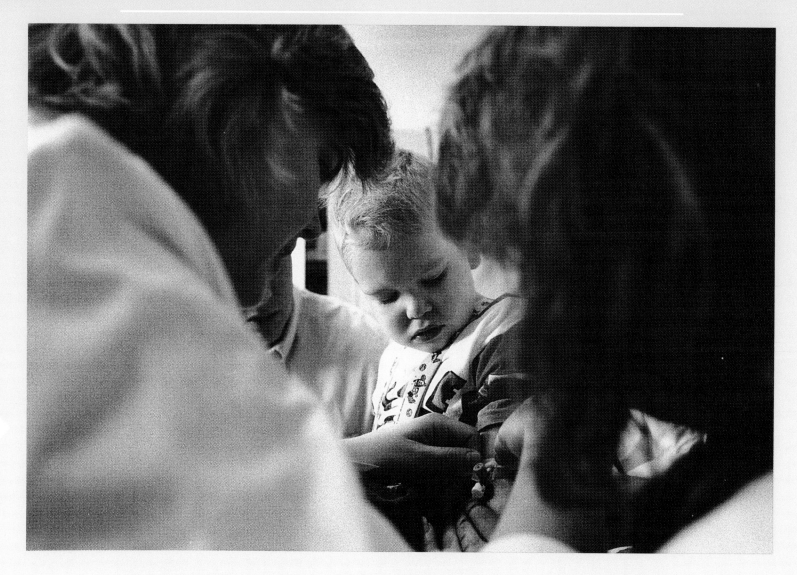

Today Frederick has come to the hospital with his father to get treatment. Frederick will get a bottle of medicine which will slowly drip into his body for the next twenty-four hours. First, however, the nurse must put a needle into a vein. Frederick has had so many injections that it is hard to find a new, strong vein to inject into. Frederick gets upset, and looks pleadingly at his father. At last the nurse finds a vein. Frederick looks up and says, 'Now the needle and the bottle are in place.' Frederick must rest now so he doesn't get a bad headache and nausea.

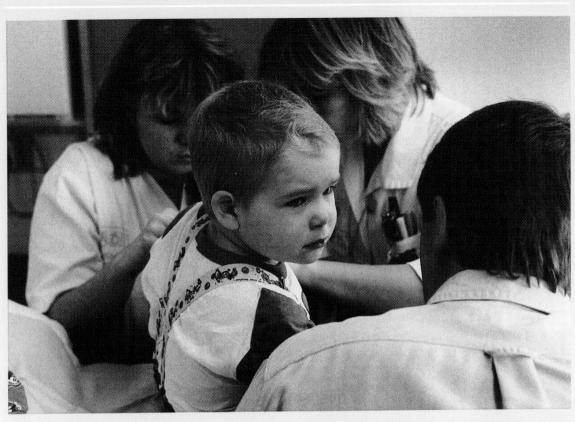

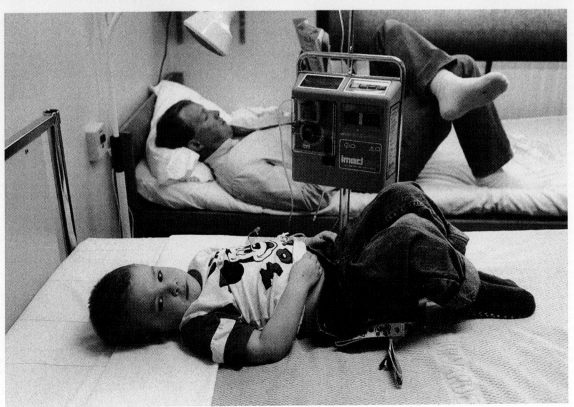

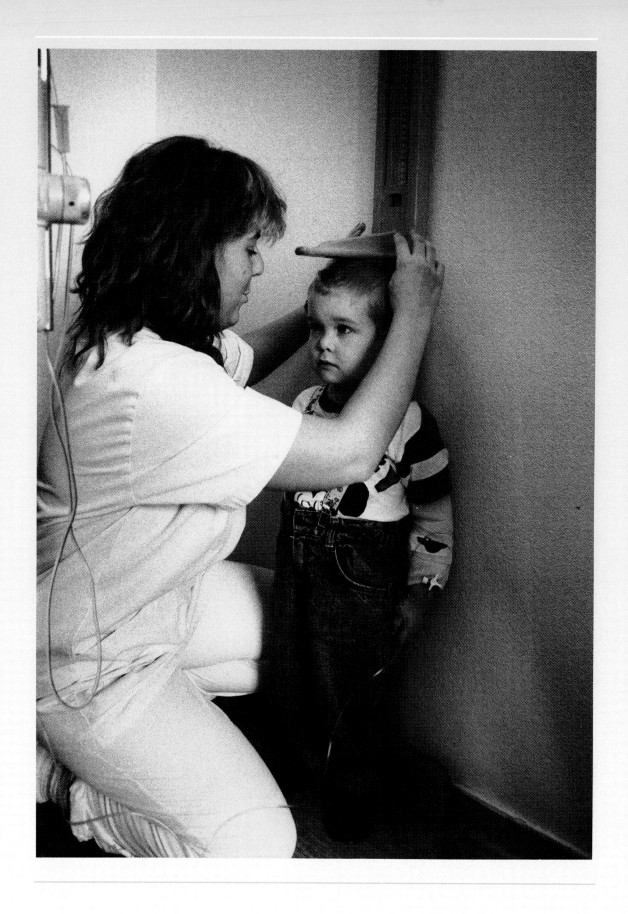

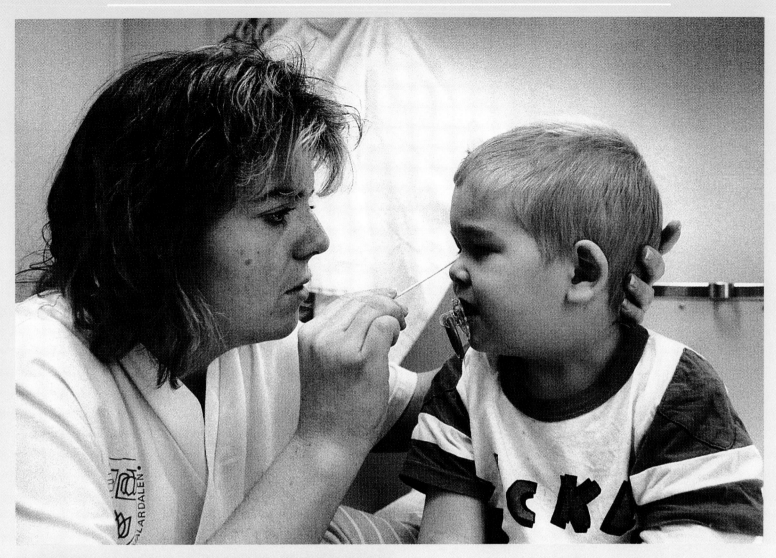

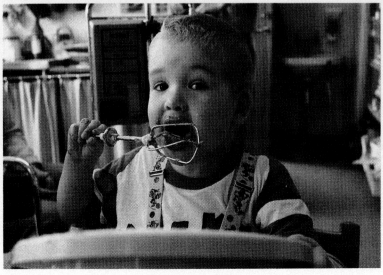

Marika, a children's nurse, calls for Frederick. 'Come here, Frederick! We have to check your weight and height to see how you've grown. Then we have to clean your eyes.' Frederick often gets infections in his eyes and ears because of the disease and the treatments. Later on, Frederick wants to go to play therapy to bake a cake, but most of all he wants to lick the mixing bowl clean.

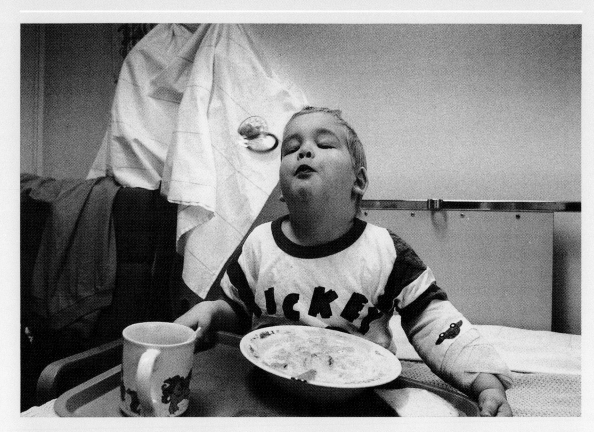

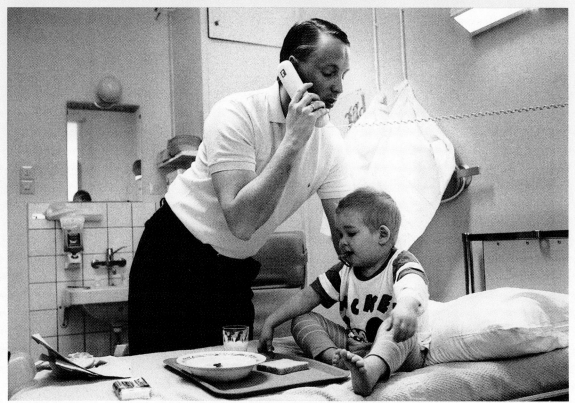

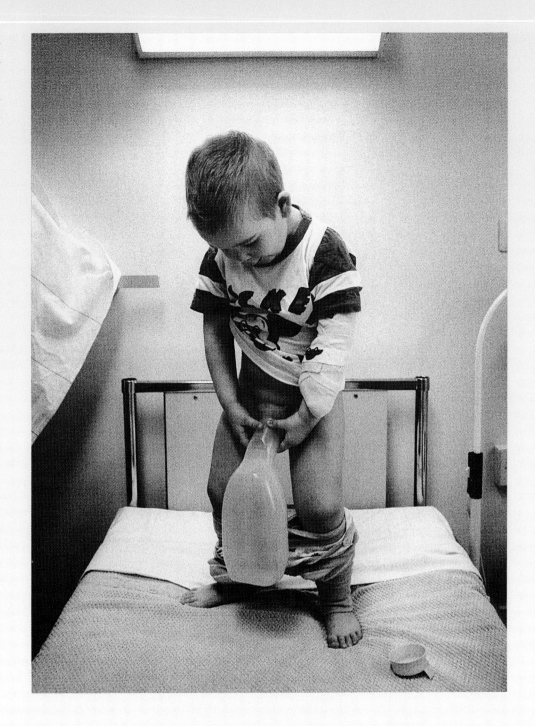

When Frederick wakes up this morning, he asks for oatmeal and milk. His father makes it for him in a kitchen down the corridor. Frederick spits out his dummy and eats a few bites, but he has lost his appetite. Suddenly, he shouts, 'Stop talking on the telephone! I have got to have the bottle to pee.' All that Frederick drinks is measured and so is his urine. Frederick knows that. He has learned a lot after so many times at the hospital.

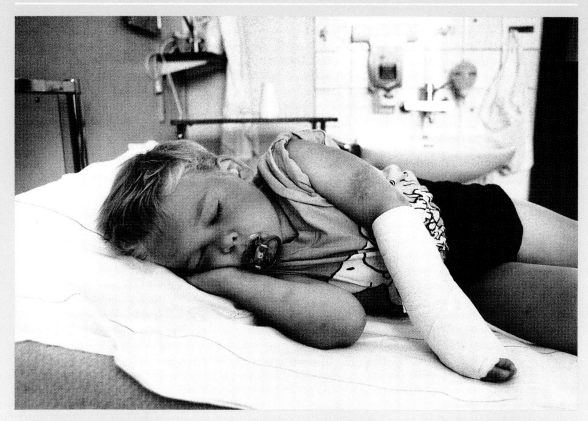

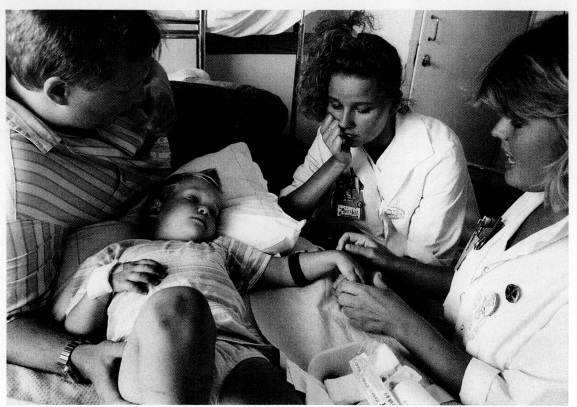

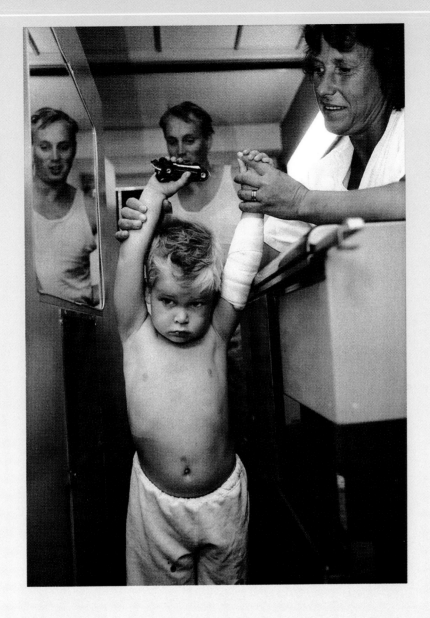

It's summer holiday time. Frederick and his family were to leave today for their summer cottage in northern Sweden. But this morning Frederick woke up and his nose was bleeding badly. The whole family has gone to the hospital instead. The nurses take care of him at once and take some blood samples. The doctor comes to the room to examine Frederick. He listens to his heart and lungs. Frederick gets some treatments and a blood transfusion, and soon his nose stops bleeding. He falls asleep. He feels much better, but the doctor has to take some X-rays of his lungs to see if Frederick has pneumonia. Frederick must stay at the hospital as long as he is sick with a cold because his nose might start bleeding again. So Frederick and his family cannot go on holiday now. Maybe they can go in the autumn instead.

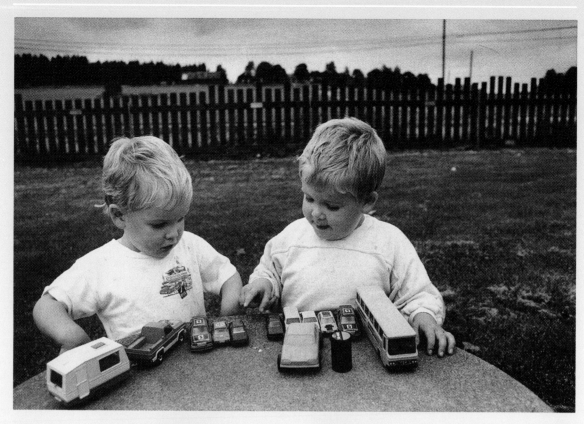

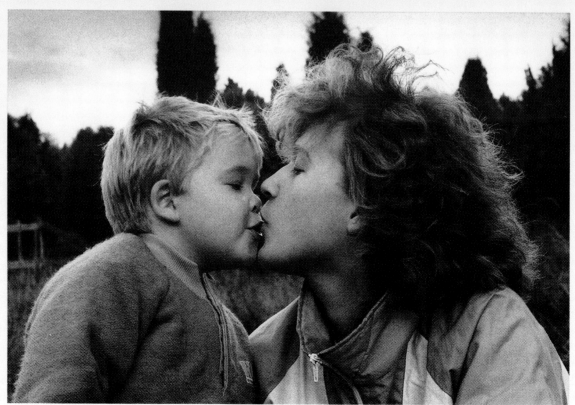

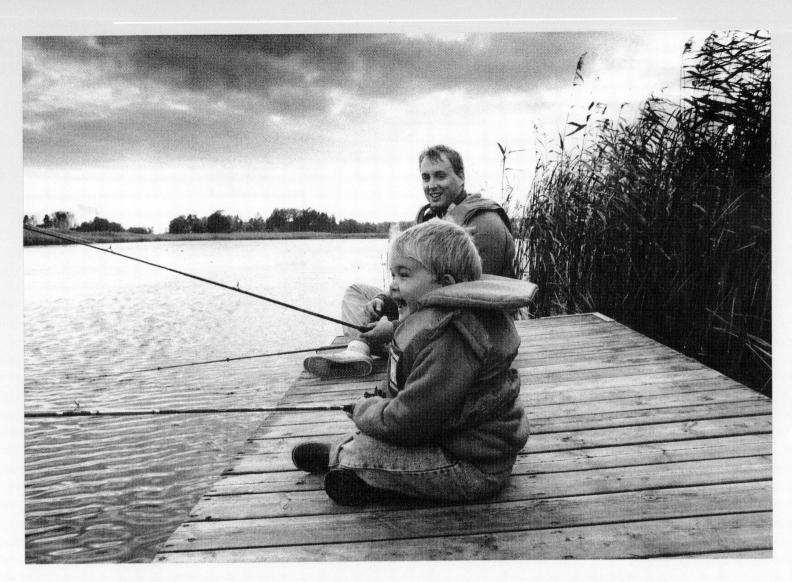

Frederick and his brother love to play with cars before dinner. Today it is Friday, which means chicken and lemonade. After dinner the boys and their father go fishing at a small lake nearby. Before they leave, Frederick's Mum gets a big hug and a kiss. Down at the small bridge it is a little windy, but Frederick likes the wind. He even gets a bite, but nothing is there. 'It was just a bottom bite,' he laughs. 'We will probably not get many fish, maybe not even one today.'

For more than a year, Frederick has endured a very difficult course of treatment. He has almost two more years to go of pills, tests, and examinations. If he does not get new symptoms, no other treatment will be needed. Frederick's parents hope that everything will go well and that he will be cured. But they know that they have no guarantee. They plan for just one day at a time.

QUESTIONS FROM CHILDREN ABOUT LEUKAEMIA AND OTHER FORMS OF CANCER

*A*sking *questions about cancer is hard. We are often too afraid of the answer to ask the question. But knowing how cancer works and how it can be treated, especially in children, may make you feel more comfortable. Here are some answers to questions children have asked. Maybe you have wondered, too.*

What is cancer?

Simply put, cancer is the presence of growing, harmful cells. Think of the body as a machine made up of working parts. The working parts of the human machine are cells. Each cell belongs in a certain place and has a job to do. If the machine is going to work well, all cells must do their job.

Cancer cells are different from normal cells in the body because they have no job to do. They only reproduce themselves and destroy normal cells. By destroying normal cells, they destroy the body's ability to operate as a good machine.

What causes cancer?

Scientists know what causes some cancers: certain chemicals, radiation, some viruses, and smoking. But cancer comes in over 100 forms. And the causes of most of these are still unknown.

What is leukaemia?

Leukaemia is a form of cancer. The disease is rooted in the tissues that make blood. The blood of a person with leukaemia contains too many abnormal white blood cells. Eventually, these abnormal white blood cells prevent the bone marrow, which produces blood cells, from making the necessary number of red blood cells, white blood cells, and platelets that make up normal blood.

The effect is this: Too few red blood cells make a person tired and weak; too few normal white blood cells allow infections to take over the body; too few platelets cause haemorrhaging, like nosebleeds and internal bleeding.

What are the signs that a person has leukaemia?

People with leukaemia may seem at first to have the flu or a very bad cold that won't go away. They will be tired and pale. They will lose weight because they have no appetite. Fevers, sweating at night, and pain in the bones and joints will make them feel sick in the same ways that flu can. But other symptoms are not like flu or any other diseases except leukaemia. These include swollen gums, red skin blotches, frequent bruises, and nosebleeds. An examination may show anaemia, enlarged lymph nodes, and an enlarged spleen and liver. The doctor makes a definite diagnosis on the basis of a blood test and a bone-marrow test, which will show if leukaemia cells are present.

What causes leukaemia?

Leukaemia is one of the forms of cancer whose cause is unknown. Cancer researchers think the answer to this question will come from studies of viruses and genes, but they cannot predict when.

Who gets leukaemia?

About 5,000 people in the United Kingdom are diagnosed with leukaemia each year. About 500 of them are children. Leukaemia is the most common form of cancer in children.

Can I catch leukaemia from someone who has it?

No. Not from the person with leukaemia nor from anything associated with him or her. Not from clothes, dishes, toilets, or kisses. Nothing. Even though scientists do not know what causes leukaemia, they do know what does not cause it. Contact with a person who has it does not cause it.

Do children with leukaemia die?

Before 1960 almost all children died within 18 months of the discovery that they had leukaemia. Today more than half of the children who get it will recover and grow up after treatment. The treatment is long and painful, but the chances of success are good.

What is the treatment for leukaemia in children?

Leukaemia is treated with chemotherapy, also called drug therapy. The purpose of chemotherapy is to destroy most cells in the bone marrow, both normal and abnormal. Because normal cells grow faster than leukaemia cells, the goal is to kill all the cells and let the normal cells reclaim the bone marrow as they grow back. Each of the two to five drugs used attacks the leukaemia cells in a specific way. The main course of treatment takes about six weeks.

What are the side effects of chemotherapy?

Chemotherapy is poison that kills the cancer cells. The drugs travel through the blood and attack the whole body. Patients suffer from vomiting and diarrhoea, sore mouth and throat, nausea and weakness. They lose weight. They are susceptible to infections and injuries. Other drugs reduce some of these side effects but even so, chemotherapy makes patients feel very sick.

Does chemotherapy make people lose their hair?

Yes, but it grows back. Sometimes it's a different colour, or straight when it was curly before. Most grown-ups wear wigs until their hair grows back. Some children wear wigs, too, or hats. Some aren't bothered by being bald. But most don't feel good about it and are glad when their hair grows back.

How can you know someone is cured?

Throughout the treatment, doctors will do tests that will show if cancer cells are still in the blood. When the treatment is successful, no signs of leukaemia will show. The patient is considered to be free of cancer.

Is remission the end of leukaemia and treatment?

It can mean the end of the leukaemia. But to be sure, the treatment continues, although less frequently. The therapy may last four years, even in children who seem cured, who have had no relapses. Patients are considered cured if they remain in remission for five years. Relapses after that are rare. Over half of the children with leukaemia will be cured.

What happens if the chemotherapy does not kill the cancer cells or if they return?

Patients who do not remain in remission for five years receive more chemotherapy. The prognosis for them is not encouraging. They may continue to have remissions, periods free of cancer, but they will probably keep getting shorter. Chemotherapy may not be as effective in killing the leukaemia cells.

If chemotherapy fails to produce remission, doctors will, in some cases, perform bone-marrow transplants. This is not a procedure available to all patients. First a suitable source of bone marrow must be found. Bone marrow withdrawn from the patient when in remission is the best source because the body will not reject its own bone marrow. If the patient has had no remissions, the only possible source is a brother or sister whose blood matches in specific ways.

But before the new marrow is transplanted, the patient's own marrow must be destroyed with drugs. This means that if the body rejects the new marrow from the sibling and its own marrow is destroyed, the patient will die. So this makes the procedure very risky when the marrow is taken from a sibling rather than the patient.

THINGS TO DO AND THINK ABOUT

You don't have to be a doctor to do something about cancer. You can contribute your energy and your ideas to help someone else. You can make new friends. Or help keep yourself or others from getting cancer.

1. Contact the children's ward of a hospital near where you live. See if you can strike up a friendship with another child by phone or as a pen pal. Probably you won't be able to visit at the hospital, but you can exchange pictures and talk and write until your friend goes home. Then, who knows?

2. Hospitals and hospices need toys and books for the children who stay there. Call to see what they can use and go through your belongings to find things you no longer use. Pick out things that are clean and have all the parts they need to work.

Think about sponsoring a toy-and-book drive with a club you belong to or with your class.

3. Find out from your hospital where families of sick children stay when they come from out of town to visit their child. A child whose brother or sister is in the hospital could become a good friend.

4. Learn what you can do to help yourself and your family lower your chances of getting cancer. Find out about the dangers of food, smoking, and pollution.

FOR MORE INFORMATION —
PLACES TO WRITE, PEOPLE TO CONTACT

The people at the organizations below may be able to send you free information about leukaemia if you write to them. When you write, tell them the reason for your interest so they can send what will be most useful to you.

Leukaemia Research Fund
43 Great Ormond Street
London WC1N 3JJ

Leukaemia Society
P.O. Box 82
Exeter
Devon EX2 5DP

Marie Curie Memorial Foundation
28 Belgrave Square
London SW1X 8QG

National Society for Cancer Relief
Michael Sobell House
30 Dorset Square
London NW1 6QL

MORE BOOKS FOR CHILDREN ABOUT CANCER

Here are some more books about children and cancer. All of these books, except the Puffin Storybook, have so far been published only in the United States.

Admission to the Feast by Gunnell Beckman (Dell, 1973)
Eric by Doris Lund (Harper & Row, 1974)

Friends Till the End by Todd Strasser (Dell, 1982)
Mama's Going to Buy You a Mockingbird by Jean Little (Puffin Storybook, Penguin, 1986)

GLOSSARY OF WORDS ABOUT
LEUKAEMIA AND ITS TREATMENT

Most words dealing with leukaemia and its treatment are scientific or medical. Their meanings are specific and some-times difficult to understand. If you need more information than the definitions below give you, ask a science teacher or your doctor.

acute lymphocytic leukaemia: the type of leukaemia that most often occurs in children, usually between the ages of two and four.

anaemia: an abnormally low number of red blood cells. A person with anaemia will be very tired.

blood transfusion: a supply of blood that is given intravenously to replace lost or damaged blood.

bone marrow: the material that fills the cavities of bones and produces blood.

cancer: a disease characterized by the growth and spread of abnormal cells. As they spread, these cells destroy normal cells. Over 100 known types exist.

cell: the basic unit of animals and plants, each with a specific function within living organisms. Cancer cells will take their place but do not do their job.

chemotherapy: treatment with chemicals, or drugs. In cancer treatment, doctors use drugs to kill the cancer cells.

clone: an exact duplicate of an original, produced by the original. Leukaemia is produced by clones of abnormal white blood cells.

coagulate: to thicken; in the case of blood, to thicken enough so that bleeding will stop.

diagnosis: medically, a doctor's opinion of what is causing a patient's problem, usually based on tests and observations.

genes: the material that determines the make-up and function of a cell and of the cells it produces.

haemorrhage: uncontrolled bleeding.

hospice: a place that cares for patients with terminal illnesses.

intravenous: injected into a vein through a needle.

malignancy: the presence of living cancer cells, indicating that a person has cancer.

microscopic: of a size too small to be seen without a microscope. A human cell is microscopic.

organism: a plant, animal, or other living being.

parasite: an organism that lives entirely off another organism, often weakening or killing that organism.

platelets: blood cells that prevent abnormal bleeding.

prognosis: medically, a doctor's opinion of how well a patient is doing or if a patient will recover.

red blood cell: scientific term, erythrocyte; the cells that deliver oxygen to the body's tissues.

remission: free of cancer cells. A long remission, usually five years, often indicates a cure. With leukaemia, remission means there are no leukaemia cells in the bone marrow and normal cells are in healthy proportion to each other.

virus: a microscopic parasite.

white blood cells: scientific term, leukocytes; blood cells whose main function is to fight off infections. Leukaemia is believed to begin with an abnormal white blood cell.

INDEX

abnormal cells 52, 53
anaemia 7, 9, 11, 14, 16

blood tests 9, 14, 20, 23, 24, 51, 53
blood transfusion 11, 16, 32, 49
blood values 24, 34
bone marrow 7, 9, 52, 53
bone-marrow transplant 53

cancer 7, 9, 52, 53
cancer ward 40
causes of cancer 52
cells 7, 13, 52
chemotherapy 7, 53
cure 7, 9, 17, 31, 51, 53

death 9, 32, 53
diagnosis 9, 52
doctors 9, 11, 13, 19, 20-21, 34, 40,
    41, 49

family support 7, 15, 16, 31, 34,
    40, 49, 51
fear 9, 11, 21, 29

genes 52

haemorrhaging 49, 52
hair, loss of 13, 23, 29, 31, 32, 53
homesickness 18

infection 7, 18, 30, 45, 52, 53
injections 13, 15, 24, 29, 31, 34,
    38, 42

leukaemia cells 7, 13, 14, 32, 52, 53

medicine 13, 19, 41, 42
microscope 13, 14

normal cells 52, 53
nurses 11, 13, 14, 18, 20, 23, 34,
    42, 45, 49

pain 7, 13, 14, 34
pills 31, 51
platelets 7, 52
playing 16, 18, 30, 37, 38, 45, 51
prognosis 53

red blood cells 7, 52
relapse 53
remission 53

siblings 30, 38, 51, 54
side effects of treatment 7, 17, 23,
    37, 41, 42, 45, 53
symptoms of leukaemia 7, 17, 18,
    19, 32, 34, 45, 49, 51, 52

toys 9, 23, 24, 37
treatment 7, 9, 13, 15, 23, 24, 27,
    29, 30, 31, 32, 34, 45, 49, 51, 53

viruses 52

white blood cells 7, 52

DATE DUE

AP 23 42			